The information in the following pages is broadly considered a truthful and accurate account of facts and as such, any inattention, use, or misuse of the information in question by the reader will render any resulting actions solely under their purview. There are no scenarios in which the publisher or the original author of this work can be in any fashion deemed liable for any hardship or damages that may befall them after undertaking information described herein.

Additionally, the information in the following pages is intended only for informational purposes and should thus be thought of as universal. As befitting its nature, it is presented without assurance regarding its prolonged validity or interim quality. Trademarks that are mentioned are done without written consent and can in no way be considered an endorsement from the trademark holder.

TABLE OF CONTENTS

BREAKFAST

Pesto Gnocchi

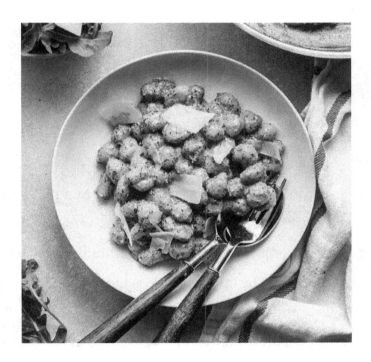

Preparation Time: 5 minutes

Cooking Time: 20 minutes

Servings: 4

Ingredients

- 1 tbsp Olive oil
- 1 Onion finely crushed
- 3 cloves garlic
- 1 sliced gnocchi jar pesto
- 1/3 cup crushed Parmesan cheese

Directions:

1. Mix the oil, onion, garlic, and gnocchi in a pan and put into the air fryer. Cook for 10 minutes, and then remove the pan and strike. Put back the pan to the air fryer and cook for 8 to 13 minutes or unless the gnocchi are lightly browned and crusty.
2. Get off the pan from the air fryer. Strike in the pesto and Parmesan cheese, and serve at once.

Nutrition: 384 Calories 25.7g Fats 28.7g Carbs 11.3g Protein

Shrimp and Grilled Cheese Sandwiches

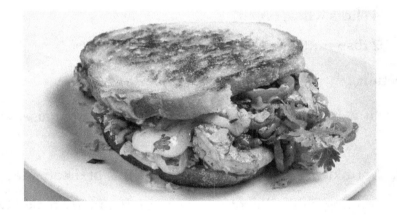

Preparation Time: 10 minutes

Cooking Time: 5 minutes

Servings: 2

Ingredients

- 1/4 cups sliced Col by Cheddar
- 1 can small shrimp,
- 3 tbsp Mayonnaise
- 4 slices wheat bread
- 2 tbsp Butter

Directions:

1. In a bowl, mix the cheese, shrimp, mayonnaise, and green onion, and properly stir.
2. Sprinkle the blend on two of the slices of bread. Have a topping with the other slices of bread to make two sandwiches. Sprinkle the sandwiches lightly with butter.
3. Bake in the air fryer for 5 to 7 minutes or unless the bread is browned and crusty and the cheese is melted. Cut in half and serve.

Nutrition: 490 Calories 65g Carbs 11g Fats 32g Proteins

Steamed Scallops with Dill

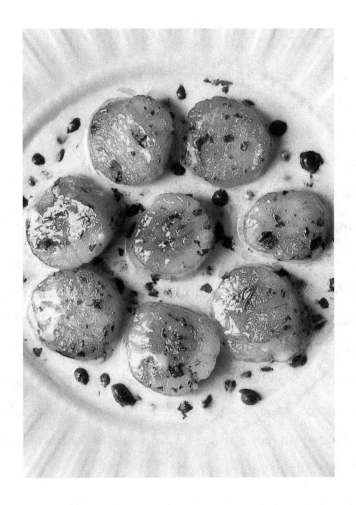

Preparation Time: 5 minutes

Cooking Time: 4 minutes

Servings: 4

Ingredients

- 1 lb. Sea Scallops
- 1 tbsp Lemon juice
- 2 tsp Olive oil
- 1 tsp Dried dill
- Pinch salt and pepper

Directions:

1. Confirm the scallops for a small muscle connected to the side, and take it off and remove it. Flip the scallops with the lemon juice, olive oil, dill, salt, and pepper. Place in to the air fryer basket.

2. Get the steam for 4 to 5 minutes, flipping the basket once while cooking time, unless the scallops are solid when tested with your finger. The inner temperature should be 62 Celsius at minimum.

Nutrition: 90 Calories 0.5g Fats 5g Carbs 4.6g Proteins

Tex-Mex Steak

Preparation Time: 25 minutes

Cooking Time: 20 minutes

Servings: 2

Ingredients

- 1 lb. Skirt steak
- 1 Chipotle pepper in adobo sauce, crushed
- 2 tbsp Adobo sauce
- 1/3 tsp Pepper
- 1/8 tsp Crushed red pepper flakes

Directions:

1. Slice the steak into four pieces and put them on a plate. In a bowl, mix the crushed chipotle pepper, adobo sauce, salt, pepper, and crushed red pepper flakes. Sprinkle over the steaks on both sides.

2. Allow the steaks stand at room temperature for at least 20 minutes, or chill up to 12 hours.

3. Cook the steaks, two at a time, in the air fryer basket for 10 minutes unless the steaks get hot. Do it again with the

rest of the steaks while the first one's rest, wrapped with foil.

4. Include the cooked steaks to the ones that have been resting and all the rest for another 5 minutes. Cut them thinly across the grain to serve.

Nutrition: 332 Calories 12g Fats 16g Proteins 36g Crabs

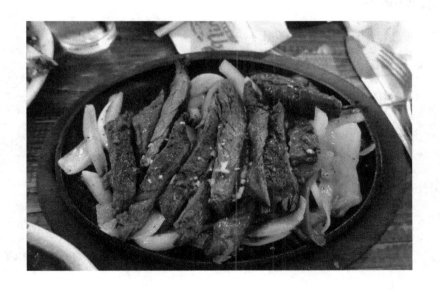

Scalloped Potatoes

Preparation Time: 5 minutes

Cooking Time: 20 minutes

Servings: 4

Ingredients

- 2 cups Refrigerated potatoes
- 2 cloves Crushed garlic
- A pinch Salt and pepper
- 3/4 cup heavy cream
- ¾ cup Heavy cream

Directions:

1. Get a layer of the potatoes, garlic, salt and pepper in a 6 by 6 2-inch pan. In a slow manner pour the cream over it.
2. Bake them for 15 minutes unless the potatoes get golden brown on the top and get soft. Check the condition and if necessary, bake for 5 minutes unless gets browned.

Nutrition: 190 Calories 7g Fats 5g Proteins 26.2g Carbs

Garlic and Sesame Carrots

Preparation Time: 5 minutes

Cooking Time: 16 minutes

Servings: 3

Ingredients

- 1 lb. Baby carrots
- 1 tbsp Sesame oil
- ½ tsp Dehydrated dill
- 6 Garlic cloves
- 2 tbsp Sesame seeds

Directions:

1. Put the baby carrots in a bowl and shake with the sesame oil, then add the dill, salt and pepper and then flip to coat properly.
2. Put the carrots in storage can of the air fryer. Roast for 8 minutes and then stir the basket once while you are cooking.
3. Include the garlic to the air fryer and roast for more 8 minutes and stir the basket while cooking unless the garlic and carrots get brown.

4. Shift all of them to a serving bowl and spread with the sesame seeds before you serve.

Nutrition: 160 Calories 11g Fats 3g Proteins 12g Carbs

Roasted Brussels Sprouts

Preparation Time: 8 minutes

Cooking Time: 20 minutes

Serving: 3

Ingredients

- 1 lb. Brussels Sprouts
- 1 tbsp Olive oil
- ½ tsp Salt
- 1/8 Teaspoon pepper
- ¼ Crushed Parmesan Cheese

Directions:

1. Clean the bases of the Brussels sprouts and draw off any stained leaves. Flip with the Olive oil, salt, and pepper, and place in the air fryer basket.
2. Bake for 20 minutes, shaking the air fryer basket two times while cooking time unless the Brussels sprouts get golden brown and crisp.
3. Shift the Brussels sprouts to a dish and flip with the Parmesan cheese. Serve at once.

Nutrition: 43.5 Calories 2.2g Fats 1.9g Protein 5.5g Carbs

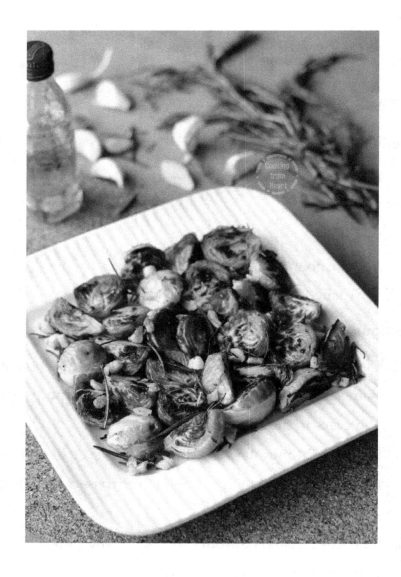

Garlic & Rosemary Breadsticks

Preparation Time: 20 minutes

Cooking Time: 30 minutes

Servings: 18

Ingredients

- ½ cup all-purpose rice flour blend
- ½ teaspoon dried rosemary, crushed
- ½ teaspoon xanthan gum
- ¼ teaspoon salt
- ½ cup water
- ¼ cup butter
- 1 small garlic clove, chopped finely
- 2 eggs
- 2 teaspoons poppy seed

Directions

1. Preheat the oven to 400 degrees F.
2. In a bowl, mix together flour blend, xanthan gum, rosemary and salt.
3. In a pan, add water, butter and garlic and bring to a boil. Reduce the heat to low. Add flour mixture and cook for

about 1 minute or until a ball is formed, stirring continuously and vigorously. Let it cool for about 5 minutes. Stir in eggs, 1 at a time and beat well after each addition until well blended.

4. In a resealable plastic bag place the dough. Seal the bag and cut a ½-inch hole from one corner. With your hands, twist bag together at the top. Now, pipe the dough into thin 8-inch strips onto an ungreased baking sheet and sprinkle with the poppy seeds.

5. Bake for 20-25 minutes. Take out from the oven and place the pan onto a wire rack to cool slightly before serving.

Nutrition: 35 Calories 3.2g Total Fat: 0.8g Protein 1g Carbs

Sesame Breadsticks

Preparation Time: 20 minutes

Cooking Time: 25 minutes

Servings: 32

Ingredients

- 2¼ teaspoons fast-acting dry yeast
- 2-2¼ cups all-purpose flour
- 2/3 cup warm water
- 1 tablespoon granulated sugar
- 1 teaspoon sea salt
- 1/3 cup olive oil
- 1 large egg white
- 1 tablespoon cold water
- 1½ teaspoons sesame seed

Directions

1. In a large bowl, place the yeast and warm water and mix until well blended. Add 1 cup of flour, sugar, 1 teaspoon of salt and ¼ cup of oil and with an electric beater, beat on medium speed until smooth. Add enough of

remaining flour, ½ cup at a time and with a wooden spoon, mix until dough a slightly sticky dough form.

2. Arrange the dough onto a lightly floured surface and with your hands, knead until dough is smooth and springy. Shape dough into a 10-inch long roll and then, cut into 32 equal sized pieces crosswise. Now, roll each piece into an 8-inch long stick. Arrange breadsticks onto greased baking sheets about 1-inch apart. on cookie sheets and coat with remaining oil. With 1 greased plastic wrap, cover each baking sheet loosely and set aside in a warm place for about 20 minutes.

3. Prepare the oven to 350 degrees and place a rack in the middle of the oven.

4. In a small bowl, place the egg white and 1 tablespoon of water and beat slightly. Coat the top of breadsticks with egg wash and sprinkle with sesame seeds.

5. Bake for about 20-25 minutes. Take out from the oven and transfer the baking sheets onto wire racks to cool slightly before serving.

Nutrition: 54 Calories 2.3g Total Fat: 1.2g Protein 7.2g Carbs

APPETIZER5 AND SIDES

Balsamic Roasted Carrots and Onions

Preparation Time: 10 minutes

Cooking Time: 50 minutes

Servings: 4-5

Ingredients:

- 2 bunches baby carrots, scrubbed, ends trimmed
- 10 small onions, peeled, halved
- 4 tbsp. brown sugar
- 1 tsp thyme
- 2 tbsp. extra virgin olive oil

Directions:

1. Preheat oven to 350 F. Line a baking tray with baking paper.
2. Place the carrots, onion, thyme and oil in a large bowl and toss until well coated. Arrange carrots and onion, in a single layer, on the baking tray. Roast for 25 minutes or until tender.
3. Sprinkle over the sugar and vinegar and toss to coat. Roast for 25-30 minutes more or until vegetables are tender and caramelized. Season with salt and pepper to taste and serve.

Nutrition: Calories: 287 Fat: 9.6g Fiber: 7g Carbs: 28.9g Protein: 9g

Spicy Carrot Slaw

Preparation Time: 10 minutes

Cooking Time: 0 minutes

Servings: 4-5

Ingredients:

- 4 carrots, shredded
- 1 apple, peeled, cored and shredded
- 2 garlic cloves, crushed
- 1/2 cup fresh dill, very finely cut
- 1 tbsp. sesame seeds
- 2 tbsp. lemon juice
- 1 tbsp. honey
- 1/2 tsp cumin
- 1/2 tsp grated ginger
- Salt and pepper, to taste

Directions:

1. Combine all ingredients in a deep salad bowl. Toss to combine, chill for 30 minutes, top with sesame seeds and serve.

Nutrition: Calories: 170 Fat: 4.5g Fiber: 7g Carbs: 22.2g Protein: 4g

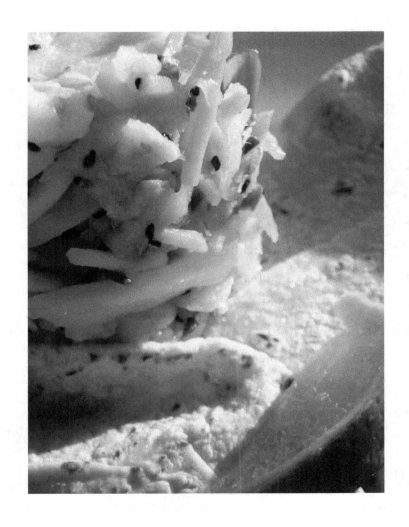

Hearty Creamy Coleslaw

Preparation Time: 10 minutes

Cooking Time: 0 minutes

Servings: 4-5

Ingredients:

- 1 head cabbage, finely shredded
- 2 carrots, finely chopped
- 2 tablespoons finely chopped onion
- ⅓ cup white sugar
- ¼ cup low–fat buttermilk
- 2 tablespoons lemon juice
- 2 teaspoon Dijon mustard
- ¼ cup Greek yogurt
- 2 tablespoons apple cider vinegar
- ¼ teaspoon celery seeds
- ½ teaspoon salt
- ¼ teaspoon ground black pepper

Directions:

1. In a large salad bowl, mix the cabbage,carrots, and onion. In a separate bowl, whisk the sugar, buttermilk, lemon juice, mustard, vinegar, celery seeds, and salt and pepper until the mixture is smooth and the sugar has dissolved. Pour the

dressing onto the cabbage mixture. Cover the bowl and refrigerate for at least 2 hours. Mix coleslaw again before serving.

Nutrition: Calories: 195 Fat: 8.7g Fiber: 4g Carbs: 19.8g Protein: 4g

Buttermilk Cast Iron Cornbread

Preparation Time: 15 minutes

Cooking Time: 25- 30 minutes

Servings: 8

Ingredients:

- 3 tablespoons butter
- 1 cup all-purpose flour
- ½ teaspoon baking soda
- 1 teaspoon baking powder
- 1 cup yellow cornmeal
- 2 large eggs
- 2 cups buttermilk
- 2 tablespoons white sugar

Directions:

1. Preheat the oven to 375°F. Place the butter in a 10–inch cast iron skillet and put in the oven while you make the batter. In a large bowl, whisk together the flour, baking soda, and baking powder. Add the cornmeal, and mix until the ingredients are well blended. In a separate bowl, whisk together the eggs and buttermilk. Add the

sugar, and blend until the sugar is dissolved. Carefully remove the cast iron skillet from the oven, and tilt the skillet until it is completely coated in butter. Pour the remaining butter into the egg mixture. Add the wet ingredients into the dry, and mix until the batter is smooth. Pour the batter into the cast iron skillet, and place it in the oven. Bake for 25–30 min., or until the cornbread is golden brown and springs back when pressed.

Nutrition: Calories: 277 Fat: 9.8g Fiber: 6.5g Carbs: 35.1g Protein: 4g

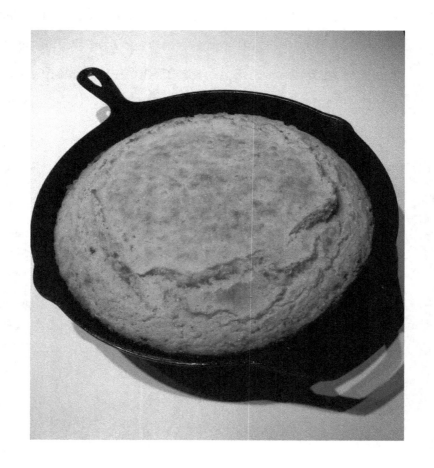

Candied Yams

Preparation Time: 7 minutes

Cooking Time: 45 minutes

Servings: 8

Ingredients:

- 2 medium jewel yams, cut into 2-inch dice
- Juice of 1 large orange
- 2 tablespoons unsalted non-hydrogenated plant-based butter
- 1½ teaspoons ground cinnamon
- ¾ teaspoon ground nutmeg
- ¼ teaspoon ground ginger
- ⅛ Teaspoon ground cloves

Directions:

1. Preheat the oven to 350°F.On a rimmed baking sheet, arrange the diced yam in a single layer. In a medium pot, combine the orange juice, butter, cinnamon, nutmeg, ginger, and cloves and cook over medium-low heat for 3 to 5 minutes, or until the ingredients come together and thicken. Pour the hot juice mixture over the yams,

turning them to make sure they are evenly coated. Transfer the baking sheet to the oven, and bake for 40 minutes, or until the yams are tender.

Nutrition: Calories: 346 Fat: 12.6g Fiber: 4.5g Carbs: 32.2g Protein: 5g

LUNCH

Pork & Bacon Parcels

Preparation Time: 5 Minutes

Cooking Time: 40 Minutes

Servings: 4

Ingredients:

- Four bacon strips
- 2 tbsp fresh parsley, chopped
- Four pork loin chops, boneless
- 1/3 cup cottage cheese
- 1 tbsp olive oil
- One onion, chopped
- 1 tbsp garlic powder
- Two tomatoes, chopped
- 1/3 cup chicken stock
- Salt and black pepper, to taste

Directions:

1. Arrange a bacon strip on top of each pork chop, divide the parsley, and cottage cheese on top.
2. Roll each pork piece and secure it with toothpicks.
3. Set a pan over medium heat and warm oil, cook the pork parcels until browned, and remove to a plate.
4. Add in the onion, and cook for 5 minutes.
5. Pour in the chicken stock and garlic powder, and cook for 3 minutes.
6. Get rid of the toothpicks from the rolls and return them to the pan.
7. Stir in black pepper, salt, parsley, and tomatoes, bring to a boil, set heat to medium-low, and cook for 25 minutes while covered. Serve.

Nutrition: Cal 433; Net Carbs 6.8g; Fat 23g; Protein 44.6g

Yummy Spareribs in Béarnaise Sauce

Preparation Time: 5 Minutes

Cooking Time: 30 Minutes

Servings: 4

Ingredients:

- 3 tbsp butter, melted
- Four egg yolks, beaten
- 2 tbsp chopped tarragon
- 2 tsp white wine vinegar
- ½ tsp onion powder
- Salt and black pepper to taste
- 4 tbsp butter
- 2 lb. spareribs, divided into 16

Directions:

1. In a bowl, whisk butter gradually into the egg yolks until evenly mixed.
2. In another bowl, combine tarragon, white wine vinegar, and onion powder.
3. Mix into the egg mixture and season with salt and black pepper; set aside.

---

4. Melt the butter in a skillet over medium heat. Season the spareribs on both sides with salt and pepper.

5. Cook in the butter on both sides until brown with a crust, minutes.

6. Divide the spareribs between plates and serve with béarnaise sauce to the side and some braised asparagus.

Nutrition: Cal 878; Net Carbs 1g; Fat 78g; Protein 41g

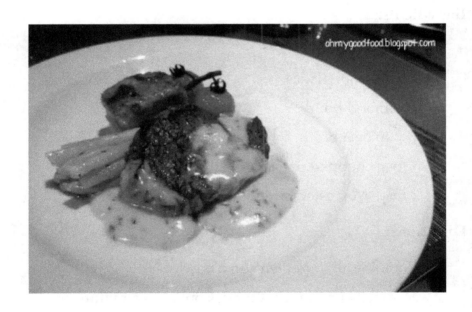

Salisbury Steak

Preparation Time: 5 Minutes

Cooking Time: 25 Minutes

Servings: 6

Ingredients:

- 2 pounds ground beef
- 1 tbsp onion flakes
- ¾ almond flour
- ¼ cup beef broth
- 1 tbsp chopped parsley
- 1 tbsp Worcestershire sauce

Directions:

1. Combine all ingredients in a bowl.
2. Mix well and make six patties out of the mixture.
3. Arrange on a lined baking sheet.
4. Bake at 375 F for about minutes. Serve.

Nutrition: Cal 354; Net Carbs 2.5g; Fat 28g; Protein 27g

Delicious Pork Stew

Preparation Time: 5 Minutes

Cooking Time: 1 Hour and 20 Minutes

Servings: 12

Ingredients:

- Two tablespoons coconut oil
- 4 pounds pork, cubed
- Salt and black pepper to the taste
- Two tablespoons ghee
- Three garlic cloves, minced
- ¾ cup beef stock
- ¾ cup apple cider vinegar
- Three carrots, chopped
- One cabbage head, shredded
- ½ cup green onion, chopped
- 1 cup whipping cream

Directions:

1. Heat a pan with the ghee and the oil over medium-high heat, add pork and brown it for a few minutes on each side.

2. Add vinegar and stock, stir well and bring to a simmer.

3. Add cabbage, garlic, salt and pepper, stir, cover, and cook for 1 hour.

4. Add carrots and green onions, stir and cook for 15 minutes more.

5. Add whipping cream, stir for 1 minute, divide between plates and serve.

6. **Enjoy!**

Nutrition: Calories 400 Fat 25 Fiber 3 Carbs 6 Protein 43

Creamy Pork Marsala

Preparation Time: 5 Minutes

Cooking Time: 30 Minutes

Servings: 4

Ingredients:

- 4 (4-ounce) boneless pork cutlets
- Salt
- Freshly ground black pepper
- Four tablespoons butter
- 8 ounces sliced mushrooms
- 4 ounces prosciutto, chopped
- One garlic clove, minced
- ½ cup Marsala cooking wine
- *½ cup* Bone Broth
- One teaspoon chopped fresh thyme
- ½ teaspoon xanthan or guar gum,
- Chopped fresh parsley for garnish

Directions:

1. Sprinkle the cutlets with pepper and salt.

2. Heat a large frypan with medium-high heat and melt two tablespoons of butter. Add the cutlets, then cook for at least 5 minutes on each side until cooked completely. Take away the cutlets from the skillet.

3. Lessen the heat to medium-low and add the remaining two tablespoons of butter. Add the mushrooms, prosciutto, garlic, and cook, frequently stirring, until the mushrooms brown, about 5 minutes.

4. Add the wine, bone broth, and thyme.

5. Cook for around 15 minutes until the sauce thickens. Add the xanthan gum to thicken the sauce even more. Put the pork back in the skillet and raise the heat to medium-high. Cook until the cutlets are heated through.

6. Serve garnished with parsley.

Nutrition: Calories: 339 Total Fat: 19g Protein: 36g Total Carbs: 6g 6g

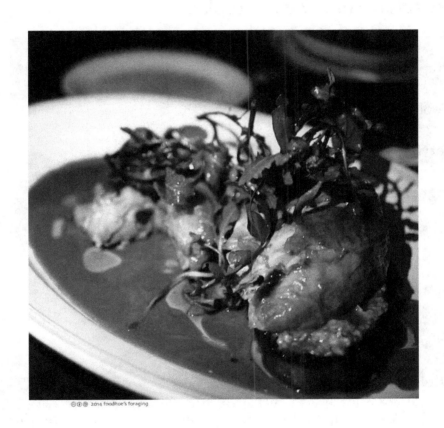

©①② 2014 foodhoe's foraging

DINNER

Roasted Turkey with Apples

Preparation Time: 10 minutes

Cooking Time: 25 minutes

Serving: 2

Ingredients

- 2 Turkey escallops
- 1 tbsp Vegetable oil
- ¼ cup Maple syrup
- 1 Green apple
- 2 tbsp Concentrated chicken broth

Directions:

1. Peel the apple from the skin and remove the core. Cut into thin slices. In a deep skillet, heat the vegetable oil over medium heat. Spread the meat and fry on both sides until cooked and a light brown crust appears.

2. Add apples and fry over light heat in a skillet, then add maple syrup and broth. Cook until apples are soft. Put the turkey on the plates, lay the apples on top, and pour the sauce.

Nutrition: 1191 Calories 38.8g Proteins 95g Fats 45g Carbohydrates

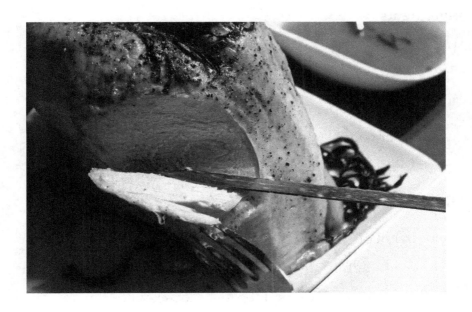

Chicken Fajitas

Preparation Time: 10 minutes

Cooking Time: 20 minutes

Serving: 4

Ingredients

- 3 Sweet pepper
- 35 oz. Chicken fillet
- 4 Chili pepper
- 2 Canned Beans
- Vegetable oil

Directions

1. In hot oil, fry slices of bell pepper. Add the diced chicken fillet, lightly fry, and add salt. Add chopped chili peppers and canned beans. Cover with the lid and simmer until tender for 10 minutes.
2. Serve with sour cream.

Nutrition: 1191 Calories 38g Proteins 91g Fats 42g Carbohydrates

Tonkatsu

Preparation Time: 15 minutes

Cooking Time: 15 minutes

Serving: 1

Ingredients

- 3.5 oz. Pork
- 0.5 oz. Ground crumbs
- 0.17 oz. Wheat flour
- 1 Chicken egg

Directions:

1. Cut the meat into thin slices. Roll each piece in flour, then roll it in a slightly beaten egg, and after in breadcrumbs. Fry in well-heated oil until tender and golden brown.

Nutrition: 305 Calories 28g Proteins 14g Fats 15g Carbohydrates

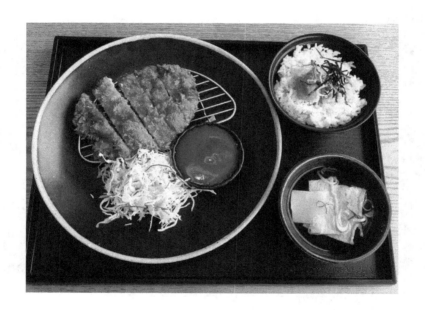

Ginger Meat

Preparation time: 5 minutes

Cooking Time: 35 minutes

Serving: 2

Ingredients:

- 14 oz. Veal
- 0.7 oz. Butter
- 2 tbsp Whole grain mustard
- 0.7 oz Fresh ginger
- Wheat flour to taste

Directions:

1. Melt the butter in a pan. Cut the ginger and toss into the pan, reduce the heat. Add mustard. Cut the meat into strips. Throw meat into the frying pan and cook until almost ready.
2. Add flour so that the mass thickens. Cook until ready. If you want, you can add a few green onions.

Nutrition: 321 Calories 43g Proteins 15g Fats 2.7g Carbohydrates

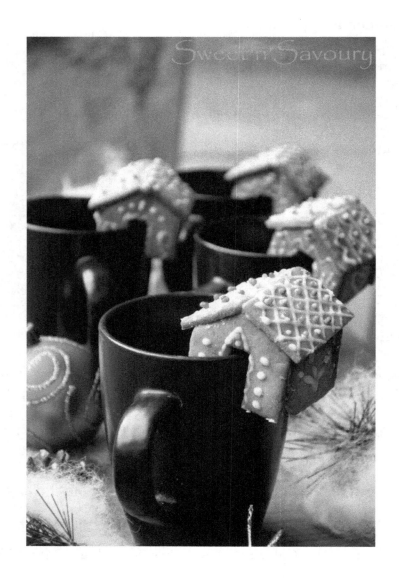

Panko-Crusted Veal Chops with Sorrel Cream

Preparation Time: 25 minutes

Cooking Time: 55 minutes

Servings: 4

Ingredients

- 1 cup crème fraiche
- 4 ounces packed sorrel leaves (2 cups); stemmed, leaves sliced into ⅓" strips
- 1 tablespoon lemon juice, freshly squeezed
- 2 large eggs
- All-purpose flour, for dredging
- 1 ½ cups Panko breadcrumbs
- 1 tablespoon milk
- Four 1" thick veal rib chops
- 3 tablespoons extra-virgin olive oil
- Zest of 1 lemon, finely grated
- 3 tablespoons vegetable oil
- Freshly ground black pepper & salt to taste

Directions

1. Preheat oven to 350 F. Over moderately low heat in a small saucepan; bring the crème fraiche to a simmer for 12 to 15 minutes, until decreased to ½ cup. Stir in the lemon juice and sorrel leaves; let simmer for 5 more minutes, until the sorrel melts into the sauce. Season the sauce with pepper and salt; remove the pan from heat.

2. Put the flour in a shallow bowl. Beat the eggs with the milk in a separate shallow bowl. Toss the panko with the lemon zest in a third shallow bowl. Season the veal chops with pepper and salt; dredge them in the flour; shaking off the excess flour then dip them into the egg mixture; let the excess to drip off. Coat the veal chops with panko, pressing to help the crumbs to adhere.

3. Now, heat the vegetable oil with olive oil over moderate high heat in a large skillet until it starts shimmering. Add 2 of the veal chops into the hot skillet & cook for 2 to 3 minutes, until browned & crisp. Decrease the heat to moderate, turn the veal chops over & cook for 2 more minutes, until browned & crisp. Transfer the veal chops to a large rimmed baking sheet. Repeat with the leftover chops.

4. Bake in the preheated oven for 12 to 15 minutes, turning them once. Gently re-warm the sorrel cream over low

heat. Place the veal chops on four plates, spoon the sorrel cream over the top; serve immediately & enjoy.

Nutrition: 374 calories 12.1g fats 3.7g fiber

Sautéed Pork and Tomato Stew

Preparation Time: 45 minutes

Cooking Time: 55 minutes

Servings: 8

Ingredients

- 2 pounds roughly chopped flat-leaf parsley, plus more for garnish
- 1 ½ pounds boneless pork shoulder
- 12 'Principe Borghese' tomatoes
- 2 ½ pounds shell beans, fresh
- 1 ½ medium onions
- 2 tablespoon flat-leaf parsley, roughly chopped
- 1 ½ leeks
- 15 garlic cloves
- ¾ cup red wine
- 6 sprigs of fresh oregano
- ¾ pound green beans
- 8 slice of country bread
- ¼ teaspoon cayenne pepper, plus more to taste
- 3 tablespoon olive oil
- Freshly ground pepper & salt to taste

Directions

1. Preheat oven to 375 F. Spread the tomatoes on 2 baking pans lined with parchment & sprinkle with 1 teaspoon of salt. Roast in the preheated oven for 40 minutes. Let cool and then transfer to a clean, cutting board & chop it roughly; set aside until ready to use.

2. In the meantime, combine pork together with 6 tablespoons parsley & minced garlic in a large bowl; let stand for half an hour.

3. Now, heat 1½ tablespoons of olive oil over low heat in a large pot until hot. Once done; add in the onions followed by the leeks & sliced garlic' cook until the onions are soft, for 10 to 12 minutes, stirring occasionally. Add in the red wine; raise the heat to high and continue to cook for 6 to 8 more minutes, until the liquid is reduced by half. Add in the leftover parsley, shell beans, oregano & water (enough to cover by a quarter of an inch). Bring everything together to a boil and then decrease the heat to a simmer; cook for 10 more minutes, uncovered. Add green beans, cayenne & 1½ teaspoons salt; continue to simmer for 12 to 15 minutes, until the beans are tender. Feel free to add more of cayenne and salt, if required. Set aside & keep warm.

4. Over high heat in a large skillet, heat the leftover olive oil for 2 to 3 minutes, until it just begins to smoke. Add in the pork mixture & sauté for 4 to 5 minutes, until cooked through, stirring frequently. Add in the reserved tomatoes & season with salt. Transfer the tomato-pork mixture to the reserved bean mixture; give the ingredients a good stir until combined well. Ladle into shallow bowls & garnish with fresh parsley. Serve with bread slices and enjoy.

Nutrition: 341 calories 12.4g fats 4.8g fiber

Best Ever Sausage with Peppers, Onions, and Beer

Preparation Time: 25 minutes

Cooking Time: 35 minutes

Servings: 6

Ingredients

- 3 pounds Italian sausage links
- 2 green bell peppers, sliced
- 3 red bell peppers, sliced
- 2 red onions, large, sliced
- 3 garlic cloves, chopped
- 2 bottles beer (12 fluid ounce)
- 3 tablespoons fresh oregano, chopped
- 1 can tomato paste (6 ounce)
- 3 tablespoons fresh cilantro, chopped
- 2 tablespoons hot sauce
- 3 tablespoon olive oil
- Pepper & salt to taste

Directions

1. Over medium high heat in a large, heavy skillet; heat the olive oil. Once hot; add & cook the sausage until all sides turn brown. Remove the sausage from pan & set aside until ready to use.

2. Deglaze the pan by pouring a bottle of beer, scraping up any blackened bits from the bottom. Place the green peppers, red peppers, garlic and onions in the pan. Stir in the leftover beer & tomato paste. Season with hot sauce, cilantro, oregano, pepper and salt.

3. Cover & let simmer for a couple of minutes, until peppers and onions are tender. Slice the sausages into bite-sized pieces & add to the peppers. Cover & let simmer until the sausage is cooked through.

Nutrition: 381 calories 11.9g fats 4g fiber

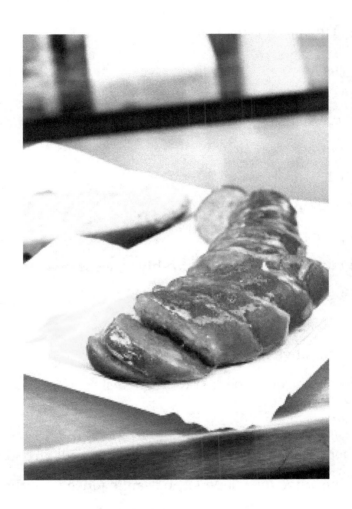

Grilled Skirt Steak with Red Wine Chimichurri

Preparation Time: 15 minutes

Cooking Time: 20 minutes

Servings: 8

Ingredients

- 5 pounds skirt steak
- 2 jalapeños
- 3 tablespoon dry red wine
- 1 garlic clove
- 3 tablespoon lime juice, freshly squeezed
- 1 tablespoon balsamic vinegar
- 2 cup each of fresh cilantro & parsley
- ½ cup olive oil
- Freshly ground pepper & salt to taste

Directions

1. Blend parsley together with lime juice, cilantro, dry red wine, olive oil, jalapeños, balsamic vinegar, garlic clove and 2 tablespoons of water in a blender. Season with salt to taste.

2. Heat your grill over high heat. Season the steaks with pepper and salt. Grill for 6 minutes per side for medium and 4 minutes for medium-rare, until you get your desired doneness. Let rest for 10 minutes; serve with the prepared sauce and enjoy.

Nutrition: 359 calories 12.7g fats 4.8g fiber

SOUP AND STEWS

Best Cream of Broccoli and Potato Soup

Preparation Time: 15 minutes

Cooking Time: 25 minutes

Servings: 3-4

Ingredients

- tablespoons butter
- 1 onion, chopped
- cloves garlic, crushed
- 1 large white potato, cubed
- 8 cups broccoli florets and stems
- salt and ground black pepper to taste
- cups chicken broth
- tablespoons butter
- tablespoons all-purpose flour
- 1 cup milk
- 1 cup heavy whipping cream

Directions:

1   In a stockpot, heat 2 tablespoons of butter over medium heat; stir and cook garlic and onion in the heated butter for 8-10 minutes until soft. Add broccoli stems and potato, liberally season with pepper and salt. Add broth to the potato mixture; put a cover on and simmer for 10 minutes until the potatoes are tender.

2   Stir into the soup with broccoli florets and simmer for 5 minutes the broccoli is soft. Using an immersion blender, blend the soup until smooth.

3   In a small saucepan, heat 3 tablespoons of butter over medium heat; stir heavy cream, milk, and flour into the heated butter. Use pepper and salt to season. Stir the milk mixture for 5 minutes until thickened and bubbling. Stir the thickened milk mixture into the soup until blended; adjust the amount of pepper and salt.

Nutrition: Calories: 364 Protein: 8.2 Total Fat: 25.9 Carbohydrate: 27.9

Best Ever Creamy Soup

Preparation Time: 15 minutes

Cooking Time 30 minutes

Servings: 4-7

Ingredients

- 1/4 cup butter
- medium onions, chopped
- heads broccoli, separated into florets
- 1 head cauliflower, separated into florets
- cups water
- pounds potatoes, peeled and cubed
- 1 (6 ounce) package baby spinach, coarsely chopped
- cubes chicken bouillon
- cups shredded Cheddar cheese

Directions:

1   In a big pot, heat butter over medium heat. Put in onions and sauté until soft. Put cauliflower and broccoli in a big pot with a minimum of 6 cups water. Boil it, and cook until the broccoli is fork-tender but remains vibrant green. Strain saving 5 cups of the liquid.

2   In a pot with the onions, add the 5 cups of saved liquid. Boil it; add bouillon cubes, spinach, and potatoes. Cook until the potatoes are soft, about 15 minutes. Take out 1/2 of the soup, and pour in a blender or food processor by small batches to puree. Put back into the pan, and mix in Cheddar cheese, cauliflower, and broccoli. Whisk it until the cheese melts, and enjoy immediately.

Nutrition: Calories: 324 Carbohydrate: 43.7 Protein: 13.1 Total Fat: 12.1

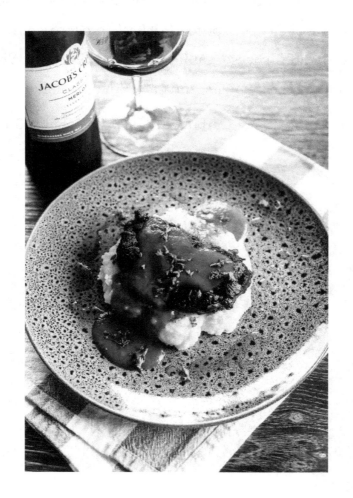

Big Game Spicy Beer Cheese Soup

Preparation Time: 25 minutes

Cooking Time: 40 minutes

Servings: 3-7

Ingredients

- tablespoons butter
- 1-tablespoon olive oil
- 1 cup finely chopped celery
- 1 cup finely chopped carrot
- 1 clove garlic, minced
- 1 (32 ounce) carton chicken stock
- (12 fluid ounce) cans or bottles American-style pale lager beer
- 1-tablespoon Worcestershire sauce
- 1-tablespoon hot pepper sauce (such as Tabasco®)
- teaspoons white pepper
- teaspoons dry mustard powder
- teaspoons onion powder
- teaspoons garlic powder
- 1 teaspoon ground cayenne pepper
- (10.75 ounce) cans condensed cream of chicken soup

- 1 (10.75 ounce) can condensed Cheddar cheese soup
- 1 (1 pound) loaf processed cheese, cubed
- 1/2 pound block pepperjack cheese, shredded
- 1/2 pound block sharp Cheddar cheese, shredded

Directions:

1   In a big soup pot/ oven, melt butter with olive oil on medium heat. Stir and cook garlic, carrots and celery for about 8 minutes until soft. Pour in cayenne pepper, garlic powder, onion powder, mustard powder, white pepper, hot pepper sauce, Worcestershire sauce, beer and chicken stock. Whisk until combined. Use a hand blender to blend mixture until smooth; boil. Lower heat to low. Simmer for 15 minutes. Mix in cheddar cheese soup and cream of chicken soup. Simmer.

2   Mix processed cheese in; let melt. When melted, mix in sharp Cheddar and pepper jack cheese, a bit at a time, letting every addition to melt into soup prior to adding the next. Simmer soup on low heat for 15-20 more minutes until cheese melts completely and flavors merge.

Nutrition: Calories: 428 Carbohydrate: 16.3 Protein: 18.6 Fat: 29.2

Brie Soup

Preparation Time: 15 minutes

Cooking Time: 40 minutes

Servings: 2-4

Ingredients

- cups chicken stock
- 1/4 cup butter
- 8 tablespoons all-purpose flour
- 12 ounces Brie cheese
- 3/8 cup white wine
- ounces julienned carrots
- 1/4 cup chopped celery
- ounces fresh mushrooms, sliced
- 1/4 cup heavy whipping cream
- Salt and pepper to taste

Directions:

1 Over low heat in a saucepan, melt butter. Put in flour and combine well, cooking until just beginning to become golden. Pour in stock and vigorously whip, cook to a boil and lower to simmer. Skim the flour and butter

and any impurities that rise to the surface and keep simmering until the veloute cooked to 2/3 of its initial quantity and the sauce becomes the heavy cream consistency.

2   Strain through a fine sieve. Over low heat, put veloute back to sauce pan and add brie cheese, slowly cook, and occasionally stir, until the cheese melted. Add veggies, wine, and lightly simmer until the veggies turn al dente. Over low heat, heat heavy cream and pour into soup. Add salt and pepper to soup to taste. Garnish with scallion or fresh chives.

Nutrition: Calories: 349 Total Fat: 27.2 Carbohydrate: 10.2 Protein: 13.5

Arborio Rice and White Bean Soup

Preparation Time: 15 minutes

Cooking Time: 20 minutes

Servings: 2-3

Ingredients

- 1-tablespoon olive oil
- garlic cloves, minced
- 3/4 cup uncooked arborio rice
- 1 carton (32 ounces) vegetable broth
- 3/4 teaspoon dried basil
- 1/2 teaspoon dried thyme
- 1/4 teaspoon dried oregano
- 1 package (16 ounces) frozen broccoli-cauliflower blend
- 1 can (15 ounces) cannellini beans, rinsed and drained
- cups fresh baby spinach
- Lemon wedges, optional

Directions:

1 Heat the oil in a big saucepan on medium heat; sauté garlic for 1 minute. Add rice; mix and cook for 2 minutes.

Mix in herbs and broth; boil. Lower the heat; simmer while covering for 10 minutes until rice is al dente.

2   Mix in beans and frozen veggies; cook while covering on medium heat for 8-10 minutes until rice is tender and heated through, occasionally mixing. Mix in spinach until wilted; serve with lemon juice if desired.

Nutrition: Calories: 303 Carbohydrate: 52g Protein: 9g Fat: 4g fat

Hearty Italian White Bean Soup

Preparation Time: 15 minutes

Cooking Time: 25 minutes

Servings: 2-4

Ingredients

- 1-tablespoon olive oil
- 1 medium potato, peeled and cut into 1/2-inch cubes
- medium carrots, chopped
- 1 medium onion, chopped
- celery ribs, chopped
- 1 medium zucchini, chopped
- 1 teaspoon finely chopped seeded jalapeno pepper
- 1 can (15-1/2 ounces) navy beans, rinsed and drained
- to 2-1/2 cups vegetable or chicken broth
- 1 can (8 ounces) tomato sauce
- tablespoons minced fresh parsley or 2 teaspoons dried parsley flakes
- 1-1/2 teaspoons minced fresh thyme or 1/2 teaspoon dried thyme

Directions:

1 Heat the oil over medium-high heat in the oven. Put in carrots and potato; cook and mix for 3 minutes. Put in jalapeno, zucchini, celery and onion; cook and mix until vegetables are crisp-tender, 3-4 minutes.

2 Mix in the rest of the ingredients; take to a boil. Lower the heat; simmer, covered, until vegetables are tender, about 12 to 15 minutes. For freezing: freeze cooled soup in freezer containers. Partially thaw overnight in the fridge to use. Heat through in a saucepan, mixing occasionally and, if needed, pouring in a little water or broth.

Nutrition: Calories: 164 Carbohydrate: 29g Protein: 8g Fat: 3g fat Fiber: 6g

VEGETABLES

Breakfast Skewers

Preparation Time: 10 minutes

Cooking Time: 10 minutes

Servings: 6

Ingredients

- 1 package (7 ounces) frozen Jones All Natural Fully Cooked Sausage Links, thawed
- 1 can (20 ounces) pineapple chunks, drained
- medium fresh mushrooms
- tablespoons butter, melted
- Maple syrup

Direction:

1 Halve the sausages and skewer alternately with mushrooms and pineapples onto five metal or water-soaked wooden skewers. Brush with butter and syrup before grilling on an open grill at medium heat, flipping

and basting until sausages are light brown and the fruits is heated through, about 8 minutes.

Nutrition: 246 calories 1g fiber 13g carbohydrate 7g protein.

Contest Winning Grilled Mushrooms

Preparation Time: 5 minutes

Cooking Time: 15 minutes

Serving: 4

Ingredients

- 1/2-pound medium fresh mushrooms
- 1/4 cup butter, melted
- 1/2 teaspoon dill weed
- 1/2 teaspoon garlic salt

Direction:

1 Thread mushrooms on 4 soaked wooden or metal skewers. Stir together garlic salt, dill, and butter, brush the mixture over the mushrooms. Grill over medium-high heat until soft, about 10-15 minutes, basting and flipping every 5 minutes.

Nutrition: 112 Calories 2g Protein 3g Fiber

Grilled Mushroom Kabobs

Preparation Time: 10 minutes

Cooking Time: 10 minutes

Serving: 4

Ingredients

- 1/2 lb. spaghetti, uncooked
- 1/4 cup BULL'S-EYE Sweet Tangy Barbecue Sauce
- cloves garlic
- 1 tsp. minced gingerroot
- 1 lb. each cremini and shiitake mushrooms

Direction:

1. Follow the package directions on how to cook the spaghetti; just omit the salt. Combine garlic, ginger, and barbecue sauce until well-blended. Thread the mushrooms alternately on the eight skewers.

2. Grill the mushrooms, turning and basting occasionally with the barbecue sauce mixture for 12 minutes. Drain the cooked spaghetti and serve it with mushrooms.

Nutrition: 300 Calories 2g Total Fat 14g Protein

Mushroom Bacon Bites

Preparation Time: 5 minutes

Cooking Time: 15 minutes

Serving: 12

Ingredients

- 24 medium fresh mushrooms
- 12 bacon strips, halved
- 1 cup barbecue sauce

Direction

1 Wrap 1 piece of bacon around each mushroom; use a toothpick to secure. Thread bacon-wrapped mushrooms onto soaked wooden or metal skewers. Brush evenly with barbecue sauce. Grill without covering for 10 to 15 minutes over indirect medium heat, turning and basting occasionally, or until mushrooms are tender and bacon is crispy.

Nutrition: 226 calories 23mg cholesterol 5g protein.

Shrimp Kabobs

Preparation Time: 5 minutes

Cooking Time: 15 minutes

Serving: 6

Ingredients

- pounds uncooked jumbo shrimp
- large onions
- 16 large fresh mushrooms
- large green peppers, cut into 1-1/2-inch pieces
- 16 cherry tomatoes

Direction:

1   Pour half cup of Italian dressing over the shrimps in a large re-sealable plastic bag. Slice 8 wedges out of each onion. Take another large re-sealable plastic bag and put in the vegetables and remaining dressing. Seal both, turn to coat, and refrigerate for 2 hours, turning from time to time. Drain both, discarding the marinade. Alternately thread the shrimp and vegetables on eight metal or pre-soaked wooden skewers. Cook kabobs in a covered grill over medium heat, or broil 4 in. from the heat, turning

occasionally, for 6 minutes or until shrimps just turn pink.

Nutrition: 150 calories 2g fat 3g fiber 13g carbohydrate 21g protein.

SNACK AND DESSERTS

Chocolate Chip Cookie Skillet

Preparation Time: 10 Minutes

Cooking Time: 25 Minutes

Servings: 8

Ingredients:

- Olive oil cooking spray, for preparing the skillet
- 1 cup almond flour
- ½ cup coconut flour
- ½ teaspoon baking soda
- 1 teaspoon salt
- ½ cup coconut oil, at room temperature
- ¼ cup sugar substitute (such as Swerve)
- 1 large egg
- One teaspoon vanilla extract
- 1 cup sugar-free chocolate chips

Directions:

1. Preheat the oven to 350 F

2. Spray a 9-inch cast-iron skillet, pie dish, or cake pan with cooking spray or grease it with coconut oil.

3. In a large bowl, beat the almond flour, coconut flour, baking soda, and salt. Add the coconut oil, sugar substitute, egg, and vanilla, and whisk until combined. Fold in the chocolate chips.

4. Pour the batter into the prepared skillet.

5. Bake it for 20 to 25 minutes, or wait until brown on the edges and gooey in the center.

6. Let sit for 5 to 10 minutes

7. Serve warm.

Nutrition: Calories: 390 Total Fat: 30g Protein: 7g Total Carbs: 25g Cholesterol: 33mg

Peanut Butter Fat Bombs

Preparation Time: 15 Minutes

Cooking Time: 1 Minute

Servings: 10

Ingredients:

- Two tablespoons coconut oil
- Two tablespoons salted butter
- ¼ cup peanut butter
- ¼ cup sugar substitute (such as Swerve)
- Two teaspoons vanilla extract
- Two tablespoons cream cheese

Directions:

1. In a medium, microwave-safe bowl, put the coconut oil, butter, peanut butter, sugar substitute, vanilla, and cream cheese. Microwave in 15-second increments, stirring in between until everything is melted and combined.

2. Pour the mixture into an ice cube tray or mini cupcake pan, and freeze for at least 4 hours.

3. Remove from the molds. Store it in an airtight vessel or a resealable plastic bag in the freezer for up to 3 months.

Nutrition: Calories: 94 Total Fat,: 9g Protein: 2g Total Carbs: 1g Cholesterol: 9mg

Roasted Cauliflower with Prosciutto, Capers, and Almonds

Preparation Time: 5 Minutes

Cooking Time: 25 Minutes

Servings: 2

Ingredients:

- 12 ounces cauliflower florets
- Two tablespoons leftover bacon grease or olive oil
- Pink Himalayan salt
- Freshly ground black pepper
- 2 ounces sliced prosciutto, torn into small pieces
- ¼ cup slivered almonds
- Two tablespoons capers
- Two tablespoons grated Parmesan cheese

Directions:

1. Preheat the oven to 400 F. Line a baking pan with a silicone baking mat or parchment paper.
2. Put the cauliflower florets in the prepared baking pan with the bacon grease and season with pink Himalayan salt and pepper. Or if you are using olive oil instead,

drizzle the cauliflower with olive oil and season with pink Himalayan salt and pepper.

3. Roast the cauliflower for 15 minutes.

4. Stir the cauliflower so all sides are coated with the bacon grease.

5. Distribute the prosciutto pieces in the pan. Then add the slivered almonds and capers. Stir to combine. Sprinkle the Parmesan cheese on top, and roast for 10 minutes more.

6. Divide between two plates, using a slotted spoon, so you don't get excess grease in the plates, and serve.

Nutrition: Calories: 288 Total Fat: 24g Carbs: 7g Fiber: 3g Protein: 14g

Buttery Slow-Cooker Mushrooms

Preparation Time: 10 Minutes

Cooking Time: 4 Hours

Servings: 2

Ingredients:

- Six tablespoons butter
- One tablespoon packaged dry ranch dressing mix
- 8 ounces fresh cremini mushrooms
- Two tablespoons grated Parmesan cheese
- One tablespoon chopped fresh flat-leaf Italian parsley

Directions:

1. With the crock insert in place, preheat the slow cooker to low.
2. Put the butter and the dry ranch dressing in the bottom of the slow cooker, and allow the butter to melt. Stir to blend the dressing mix and butter.
3. Add the mushrooms to the slow cooker, and stir to coat with the butter-dressing mixture. Sprinkle the top with the Parmesan cheese.
4. Close its lid and cook on low for 4 hours.

5. Use a slotted spoon to transfer the mushrooms to a serving dish. Top with the chopped parsley and serve.

Nutrition: Calories: 351 Total Fat: 36g Carbs: 5g Fiber: 1g Protein: 6g

Baked Zucchini Gratin

Preparation Time: 10 Minutes

Cooking Time: 25 Minutes

Servings: 2

Ingredients:

- One large zucchini, cut into ¼-inch-thick slices
- Pink Himalayan salt
- 1-ounce Brie cheese, rind trimmed off
- One tablespoon butter
- Freshly ground black pepper
- 1/3 cup shredded Gruyère cheese
- ¼ cup crushed pork rinds

Directions:

1. Salt the zucchini slices and put them in a colander in the sink for 45 minutes; the zucchini will shed much of their water.
2. Preheat the oven to 400 F.
3. When the zucchini has been "weeping" for about 30 minutes, in a small saucepan over medium-low heat, heat the Brie and butter, occasionally stirring, until the

cheese has melted and the mixture is thoroughly combined, about 2 minutes.

4. Arrange the zucchini in an 8-inch baking dish, so the zucchini slices overlap a bit—season with pepper.

5. Pour the Brie mixture over the zucchini, and top with the shredded Gruyère cheese.

6. Sprinkle the crushed pork rinds over the top.

7. Bake for about 25 minutes, until the dish is bubbling and the top is nicely browned, and serve.

Nutrition: Calories: 355 Total Fat: 25g Carbs: 5g Fiber: 2g Protein: 28g

Roasted Radishes with Brown Butter Sauce

Preparation Time: 10 Minutes

Cooking Time: 15 Minutes

Servings: 2

Ingredients:

- 2 cups halved radishes
- One tablespoon olive oil
- Pink Himalayan salt
- Freshly ground black pepper
- Two tablespoons butter
- One tablespoon chopped fresh flat-leaf Italian parsley

Directions:

1. Preheat the oven to 450 F.
2. In a medium bowl, toss the radishes in the olive oil and season with pink Himalayan salt and pepper.
3. Spread the radishes on a baking sheet in a single layer— roast for 15 minutes, stirring halfway through.
4. Meanwhile, when the radishes have been roasting for about 10 minutes, in a small, light-colored saucepan over medium heat, melt the butter completely, stirring

frequently, and season with pink Himalayan salt. Wait for the butter starts to bubble and foam, continue stirring. When the bubbling diminishes a bit, the butter should be a nice nutty brown. The browning process should take about 3 minutes in total. Transfer the browned butter to a heat-safe container (I use a mug).

5. Remove the radishes from the oven, and divide them between two plates. Spoon the brown butter over the radishes, top with the chopped parsley, and serve.

Nutrition: Calories: 181 Total Fat: 19g Carbs: 4g Protein: 1g

Parmesan and Pork Rind Green Beans

Preparation Time: 5 Minutes

Cooking Time: 15 Minutes

Servings: 2

Ingredients:

- ½ pound fresh green beans
- Two tablespoons crushed pork rinds
- Two tablespoons olive oil
- One tablespoon grated Parmesan cheese
- Pink Himalayan salt
- Freshly ground black pepper

Directions:

1. Preheat the oven to 400°F.
2. In a medium bowl, blend the green beans, pork rinds, olive oil, and Parmesan cheese. Season with pink Himalayan salt and pepper, and toss until the beans are thoroughly coated.
3. Spread the bean mixture on a baking sheet in a single layer and roast for about 15 minutes. At the halfway

point, give the pan a little shake to move the beans around, or just stir them.

4. Divide the beans between two plates and serve.

Nutrition: Calories: 175 Total Fat: 15g Carbs: 8g Fiber: 3g Protein: 6g

Pesto Cauliflower Steaks

Preparation Time: 5 Minutes

Cooking Time: 20 Minutes

Servings: 2

Ingredients:

- Two tablespoons olive oil, plus more for brushing
- ½ head cauliflower
- Pink Himalayan salt
- Freshly ground black pepper
- 2 cups fresh basil leaves
- ½ cup grated Parmesan cheese
- ¼ cup almonds
- ½ cup shredded mozzarella cheese

Directions:

1. Preheat the oven to 425°F.
2. Brush a baking sheet by means of olive oil or line with a silicone baking mat.
3. To prep the cauliflower steaks, remove and discard the leaves and cut the cauliflower into 1-inch-thick slices.

You can roast the extra floret crumbles that fall off with the steaks.

4. Place the cauliflower steaks on the arranged baking sheet, and brush them with the olive oil. You want the surface just lightly coated, so it gets caramelized— season with pink Himalayan salt and pepper.

5. Roast the cauliflower steaks for 20 minutes.

6. Meanwhile, put the basil, Parmesan cheese, almonds, and two tablespoons of olive oil in a food processor (or blender) and season with pink Himalayan salt and pepper. Mix until combined.

7. Spread some pesto on top of each cauliflower steak, and top with the mozzarella cheese. Return to the oven and bake until the cheese melts, about 2 minutes.

8. Place the cauliflower steaks on two plates, and serve hot.

Nutrition: Calories: 448 Total Fat: 34g Carbs: 17 Fiber: 7g Protein: 24g

Tomato, Avocado, and Cucumber Salad

Preparation Time: 5 Minutes

Cooking Time: 0 Minutes

Servings: 2

Ingredients:

- ½ cup grape tomatoes halved
- Four small Persian cucumbers or 1 English cucumber, peeled and finely chopped
- One avocado, finely chopped
- ¼ cup crumbled feta cheese
- Two tablespoons vinaigrette salad dressing
- Pink Himalayan salt
- Freshly ground black pepper

Directions:

1. In a large bowl, blend the tomatoes, cucumbers, avocado, and feta cheese.
2. Add the vinaigrette, and season with pink Himalayan salt and pepper. Toss to combine thoroughly.
3. Divide the salad between two plates and serve.

Nutrition: Calories: 258 Total Fat: 23g Carbs: 12g Protein: 5g

Crunchy Pork Rind Zucchini Sticks

Preparation Time: 5 Minutes

Cooking Time: 25 Minutes

Servings: 2

Ingredients:

- Two medium zucchinis halved lengthwise and seeded
- ¼ cup crushed pork rinds
- ¼ cup grated Parmesan cheese
- Two garlic cloves, minced
- Two tablespoons melted butter
- Pink Himalayan salt
- Freshly ground black pepper
- Olive oil, for drizzling

Directions:

1. Preheat the oven to 400°F.
2. Place the zucchini splits cut-side up on the prepared baking sheet.
3. Toss the pork rinds, Parmesan cheese, garlic, melted butter, and season with pink Himalayan salt and pepper in a bowl. Mix until well combined.

4. Spoon the pork-rind mixture onto each zucchini stick, and drizzle each with a little olive oil.

5. Bake for around 20 minutes, or wait until the topping is golden brown.

6. Switch on the broiler to finish browning the zucchini sticks, 3 to 5 minutes, and serve.

Nutrition: Calories: 231 Total Fat: 20g Carbs: 8g Fiber: 2g Protein: 9g